Doomed!

PLAGUE
THE BLACK DEATH

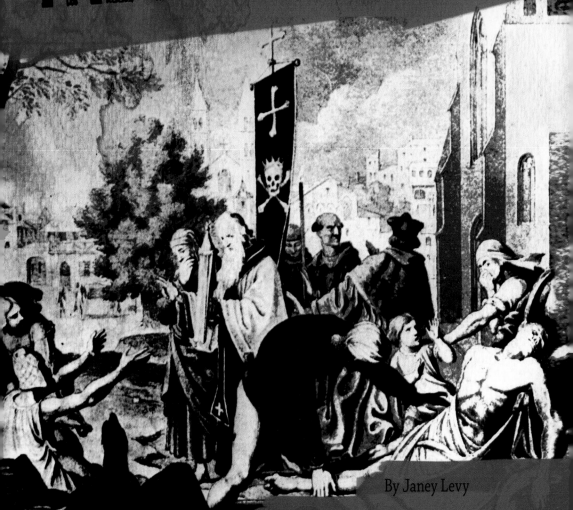

By Janey Levy

Gareth Stevens
PUBLISHING

Please visit our website, www.garethstevens.com. For a free color catalog
of all our high-quality books, call toll free 1-800-542-2595 or fax 1-877-542-2596.

Library of Congress Cataloging-in-Publication Data

Levy, Janey.
  Plague : the black death / Janey Levy.
      pages cm. — (Doomed!)
  Includes bibliographical references and index.
  ISBN 978-1-4824-2940-4 (pbk.)
  ISBN 978-1-4824-2941-1 (6 pack)
  ISBN 978-1-4824-2942-8 (library binding)
  1. Plague. 2. Black Death—Europe—History. 3. Epidemics. I. Title.
  RA644.P7L48 2016
  614.5'732094—dc23

                                        2015012144

First Edition

Published in 2016 by
Gareth Stevens Publishing
111 East 14th Street, Suite 349
New York, NY 10003

Designer: Katelyn E. Reynolds
Editor: Therese Shea

Photo credits: Cover, pp. 1, 13 Hulton Archive/Getty Images; cover, pp. 1–32
(background texture) 501room/Shutterstock.com; pp. 5, 23 Ann Ronan Pictures/
Print Collector/Getty Images; pp. 7, 18 NYPL/Science Source/Getty Images; p. 9
Andrey Bayda/Shutterstock.com; p. 11 Leemage/Universal Images Group/Getty
Images; p. 15 Master of Puppets and Alexrk2/Wikipedia.org; pp. 17, 19 DeAgostini/
Getty Images; pp. 21, 27 MOLA/Getty Images; p. 25 Photo12/UIG via Getty Images;
p. 29 Michel du Cille/The Washington Post via Getty Images.

Printed in the United States of America

CPSIA compliance information: Batch #CS15GS: For further information contact Gareth Stevens, New York, New York at 1-800-542-2595.

CONTENTS

Words in the glossary appear in **bold** type
the first time they are used in the text.

DEATH SHIPS

On a fine early October day in 1347, 12 Italian trading ships docked at Messina, Sicily. They were returning from the Black Sea, a key link in Europe's trade with China. A crowd had gathered to greet them, but the mood quickly turned to horror.

Most of the sailors on the ships were dead. Those still alive suffered high fever, **vomiting**, and severe pain. Black boils leaking blood and **pus** covered them. Alarmed officials ordered the "death ships" to leave, but it was too late. The Black Death had reached Europe, and it would kill tens of millions over the next 5 years.

What was the Black Death? Where did it come from, and how was it able to kill so many? Why couldn't its spread be stopped?

The Deadly Details

The Italian ships had been to a trading post in modern-day Ukraine that was attacked. The attacking army launched bodies of Black Death victims into the trading post, spreading the disease to the sailors.

4

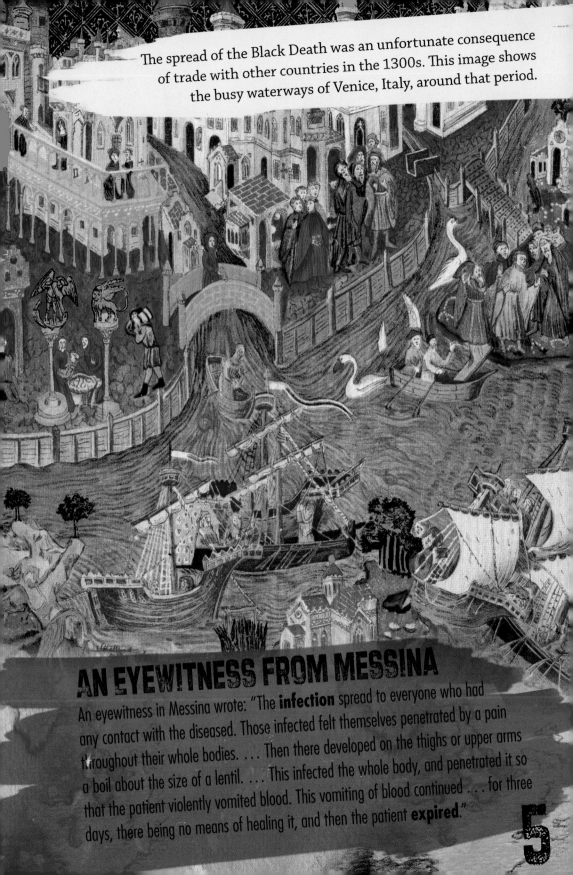

The spread of the Black Death was an unfortunate consequence of trade with other countries in the 1300s. This image shows the busy waterways of Venice, Italy, around that period.

AN EYEWITNESS FROM MESSINA

An eyewitness in Messina wrote: "The **infection** spread to everyone who had any contact with the diseased. Those infected felt themselves penetrated by a pain throughout their whole bodies. ... Then there developed on the thighs or upper arms a boil about the size of a lentil. ... This infected the whole body, and penetrated it so that the patient violently vomited blood. This vomiting of blood continued ... for three days, there being no means of healing it, and then the patient **expired**."

THE DISEASE

Today, most experts believe the Black Death was plague, which is caused by the bacterium *Yersinia pestis*. *Y. pestis* normally infects rats, which then—as now—could be found wherever people lived. It's transmitted by fleas.

Plague occurs in three equally terrible forms: bubonic, pneumonic, and septicemic. Some believe the Black Death involved more than one form. Bubonic plague is the most common form and the one transmitted by fleas. The symptoms, or signs, include high fever, aching limbs, vomiting blood, and buboes—swollen **lymph** glands in the victim's neck, armpits, and **groin**—which give this form its name. The symptoms appear about 4 days after infection, and about 60 percent of people die within about 4 days after symptoms appear.

The Deadly Details

The Black Death may have gotten its name from the black boils and buboes on victims' bodies. Or the name may have come from the Latin name for the disease: *atra mors*. *Mors* means "death," and *atra* means "terrible" or "black."

6

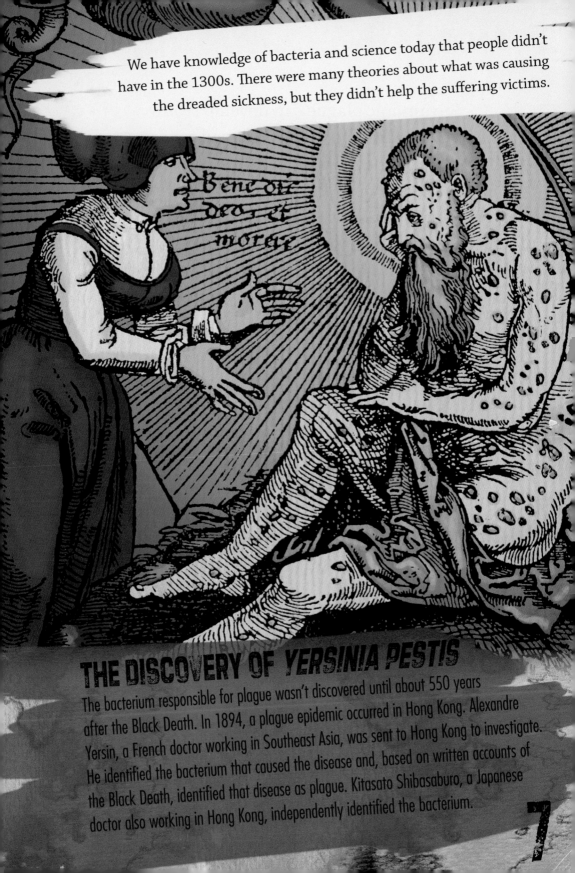

We have knowledge of bacteria and science today that people didn't have in the 1300s. There were many theories about what was causing the dreaded sickness, but they didn't help the suffering victims.

THE DISCOVERY OF *YERSINIA PESTIS*

The bacterium responsible for plague wasn't discovered until about 550 years after the Black Death. In 1894, a plague epidemic occurred in Hong Kong. Alexandre Yersin, a French doctor working in Southeast Asia, was sent to Hong Kong to investigate. He identified the bacterium that caused the disease and, based on written accounts of the Black Death, identified that disease as plague. Kitasato Shibasaburo, a Japanese doctor also working in Hong Kong, independently identified the bacterium.

Pneumonic plague can develop from bubonic plague if the bacteria spread to the lungs. It's the most serious form of the disease and the only one that can be spread from person to person, much like a cold can be spread. Symptoms include fever, headache, weakness, difficulty breathing, chest pain, cough, and bloody or watery **mucus**. Pneumonic plague is almost 100 percent fatal, and victims may die within hours of infection.

Septicemic plague attacks the blood and can develop from untreated bubonic plague. Symptoms include fever, chills, extreme weakness, stomach pain, and possibly bleeding into the skin and other organs. Skin and other tissues of the body may turn black and die, especially on fingers, toes, and the nose. Like pneumonic plague, it's almost 100 percent fatal.

The DeadLy DetaiLS

If a victim of bubonic plague lived long enough—and many didn't—their buboes would burst and spurt out pus. This was extremely painful, and accounts describe victims leaping from their bed and screaming in pain.

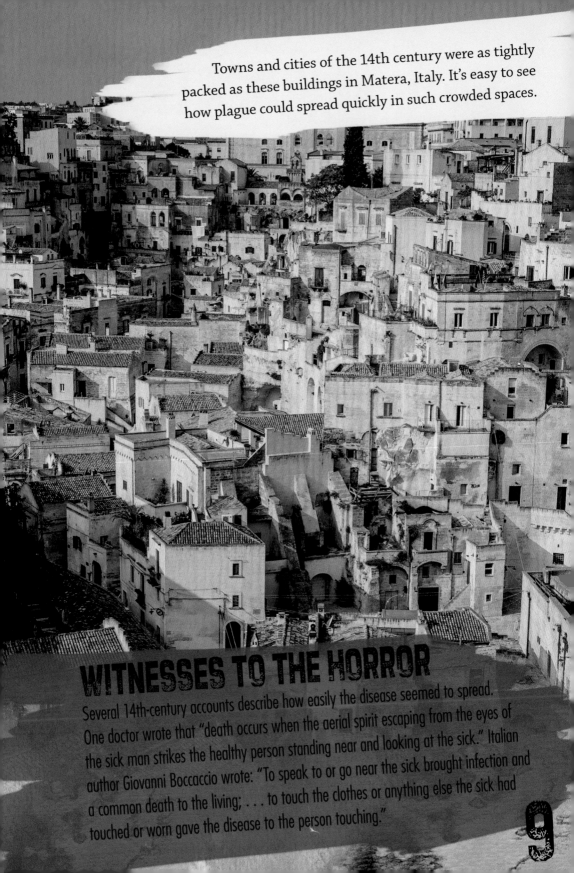

Towns and cities of the 14th century were as tightly packed as these buildings in Matera, Italy. It's easy to see how plague could spread quickly in such crowded spaces.

WITNESSES TO THE HORROR

Several 14th-century accounts describe how easily the disease seemed to spread. One doctor wrote that "death occurs when the aerial spirit escaping from the eyes of the sick man strikes the healthy person standing near and looking at the sick." Italian author Giovanni Boccaccio wrote: "To speak to or go near the sick brought infection and a common death to the living; . . . to touch the clothes or anything else the sick had touched or worn gave the disease to the person touching."

THE BLACK DEATH'S JOURNEY TO EUROPE

The Black Death erupted in the 1330s somewhere in Asia, either in China or in the region now occupied largely by Kazakhstan. It was carried west along trade routes or with the **Mongol** army. By 1346, it had reached the region of Crimea in modern-day Ukraine, where it attacked the Mongol army. It spread to the Italian trading post there and infected sailors.

From the trading post in Crimea, the spread of the Black Death followed trade routes. Ships carried it to the Mediterranean island of Cyprus in the summer of 1347. It hit the French city of Marseilles in September. As you read earlier, the Black Death reached Messina, Sicily, in October. It arrived in the Italian cities of Venice, Pisa, and Genoa in November. Escape became impossible.

The Deadly Details

The 14th century wasn't the first time plague appeared. Europe suffered a plague epidemic in the sixth century that killed millions, but the disease had been fairly quiet in the centuries since then.

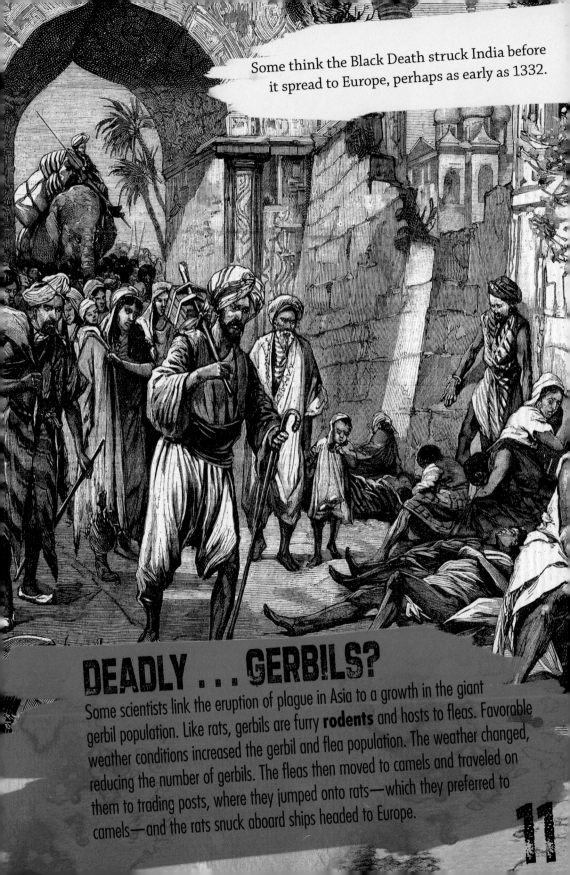

Some think the Black Death struck India before it spread to Europe, perhaps as early as 1332.

DEADLY . . . GERBILS?

Some scientists link the eruption of plague in Asia to a growth in the giant gerbil population. Like rats, gerbils are furry **rodents** and hosts to fleas. Favorable weather conditions increased the gerbil and flea population. The weather changed, reducing the number of gerbils. The fleas then moved to camels and traveled on them to trading posts, where they jumped onto rats—which they preferred to camels—and the rats snuck aboard ships headed to Europe.

11

THE BLACK DEATH SPREADS ACROSS EUROPE

Once the Black Death reached Europe, it spread with astonishing speed along trade routes. From Marseilles, France, it moved out in two directions: north along the Rhône River into the heart of Europe and southwest along the Mediterranean coast toward Spain. When it reached the city of Narbonne in its coastal journey, it again went in two directions—on toward Spain and over a land route to the commercial center of Bordeaux on the Atlantic coast.

During the spring and summer of 1348, ships from Bordeaux carried the Black Death to Spanish ports and to northern France. From northern France, the disease spread toward Paris and what are today the countries of the Netherlands and Belgium. Another ship from Bordeaux carried the Black Death to southern England. By August, it had reached London.

The Deadly Details

Carried by ships, the Black Death spread about 25 miles (40 km) per day. Over land, it spread much more slowly—about 1.2 miles (2 km) per day.

12

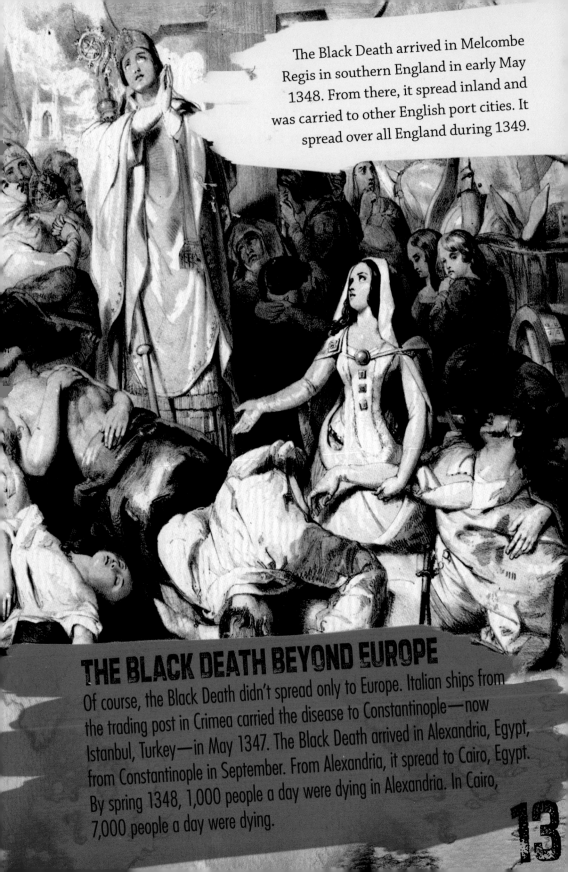

The Black Death arrived in Melcombe Regis in southern England in early May 1348. From there, it spread inland and was carried to other English port cities. It spread over all England during 1349.

THE BLACK DEATH BEYOND EUROPE

Of course, the Black Death didn't spread only to Europe. Italian ships from the trading post in Crimea carried the disease to Constantinople—now Istanbul, Turkey—in May 1347. The Black Death arrived in Alexandria, Egypt, from Constantinople in September. From Alexandria, it spread to Cairo, Egypt. By spring 1348, 1,000 people a day were dying in Alexandria. In Cairo, 7,000 people a day were dying.

13

Ships from England carried the Black Death to Oslo, Norway, in the autumn of 1348. From there, it spread inland. Another ship from England brought the disease to Bergen, Norway, in July 1349.

Oslo and Bergen were important commercial centers visited by ships from many northern European countries, and, like Marseilles, they acted as centers from which the disease spread. Ships from Norway carried the Black Death to numerous northern European cities in 1349. In spring 1350, the disease spread south into Europe's heartland and met the disease spreading north from the Rhône River.

In autumn 1351, the Black Death entered Russia. It laid waste to Moscow in 1353 and once again reached the Mongols. It had come full circle.

The Deadly Details

Finland and Iceland managed to avoid the Black Death. They had little contact with other nations and small populations, which would have made it hard for the disease to spread.

14

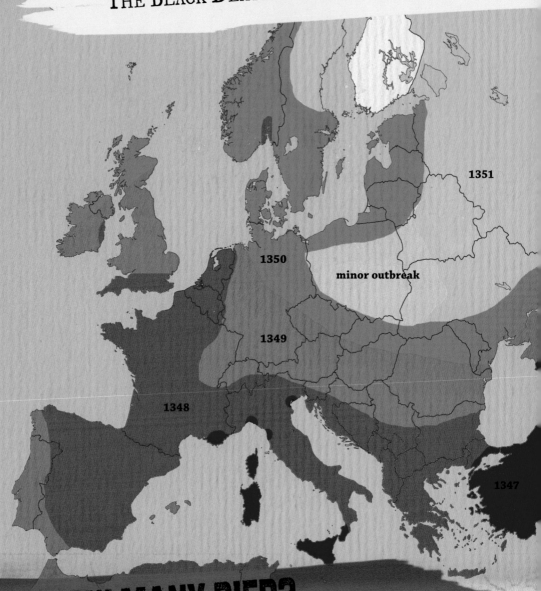

1351

1350

minor outbreak

1349

1348

1347

HOW MANY DIED?

It's difficult to say for sure how many died during the Black Death in Europe. For a long time, most experts agreed it was probably around 25 million people, or about 30 percent of the population. Recently, however, an expert has studied the records that tell about deaths, taking into account the information the records leave out about women, children, and the poor. He estimates about 50 million people, or 60 percent of the population, died!

DOOMED BY IGNORANCE AND FEAR

What did people make of the great tragedy that had come to them, and how did they deal with it? The well educated knew it was a disease, not punishment from God, but the 14th-century understanding of diseases, their causes, and their treatment was very different from the modern understanding.

The doctors at the College of Physicians in Paris, France, gave their opinion: The disease resulted from the way the planets Saturn, Jupiter, and Mars had lined up in the sign of Aquarius in 1345. This event caused hot, moist conditions, which led Earth to release poisonous vapors, called miasmas. These produced the deadly disease.

With this understanding of the cause of the Black Death, efforts to treat and control it were doomed from the start.

The Deadly Details

The Paris doctors made suggestions for avoiding the disease, such as not eating fowl, fish, pig, old beef, or olive oil. They also cautioned: "It is injurious to sleep during the daytime . . . too much exercise may be injurious. . . . Bathing is dangerous."

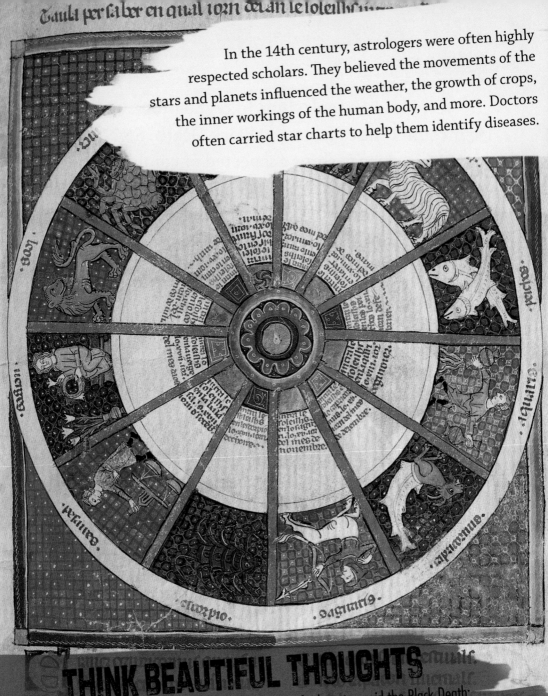

In the 14th century, astrologers were often highly respected scholars. They believed the movements of the stars and planets influenced the weather, the growth of crops, the inner workings of the human body, and more. Doctors often carried star charts to help them identify diseases.

THINK BEAUTIFUL THOUGHTS

Scholars from Italy had their own suggestions for how to avoid the Black Death: "In the first instance, no man should think of death. ... Nothing should distress him, but all his thoughts should be directed to pleasing, agreeable and delicious things. ... Beautiful landscapes, fine gardens should be visited. ... Listening to beautiful, melodious songs is wholesome. ... The contemplating of gold and silver and other precious stones is comforting to the heart."

City leaders took steps to try to protect their communities from the Black Death. Some ports turned away ships suspected of coming from infected areas. Venice, Italy, went a step further. Even ships that weren't believed to have come from infected areas were kept **isolated** for 30 days to make sure no one on board was sick.

Milan, Italy, took harsh measures to try to prevent the spread of the disease. When someone in a house was found to be infected, the house was walled up with everyone inside, the healthy as well as the sick. City leaders took a new approach in 1350. They had a "pesthouse" built outside the city walls, and all those who were sick, along with those nursing them, would be isolated there.

The Deadly Details

Other treatments doctors used included bloodletting, or cutting open blood vessels, to drain away poisons; burning fragrant herbs; and bathing patients in rosewater or vinegar.

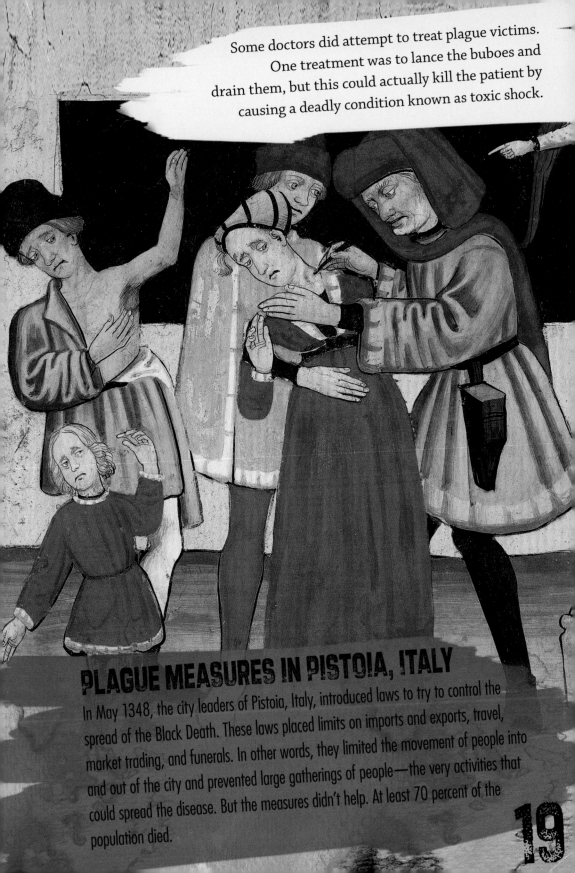

Some doctors did attempt to treat plague victims. One treatment was to lance the buboes and drain them, but this could actually kill the patient by causing a deadly condition known as toxic shock.

PLAGUE MEASURES IN PISTOIA, ITALY

In May 1348, the city leaders of Pistoia, Italy, introduced laws to try to control the spread of the Black Death. These laws placed limits on imports and exports, travel, market trading, and funerals. In other words, they limited the movement of people into and out of the city and prevented large gatherings of people—the very activities that could spread the disease. But the measures didn't help. At least 70 percent of the population died.

The general population panicked, terrified by this horrible disease. Healthy people avoided the sick. Some doctors refused to see patients. Some priests refused to attend to the dying. Shopkeepers closed their stores. Those who could afford to fled the cities for the countryside in hopes of escaping the Black Death. But they found it waiting for them, for the disease also infected cows, sheep, goats, pigs, and chickens. In fact, so many sheep died there was a wool shortage.

Italian author Boccaccio wrote how, in a desperate effort to save themselves, people abandoned their sick and dying loved ones: "brother abandoned brother, and the uncle his nephew, and the sister her brother, and very often the wife her husband." Even worse, he wrote, parents refused to care for their children.

The Deadly Details

People tried some wild "cures" for the Black Death: tying live chickens around buboes, drinks containing poisons such as mercury or arsenic, and even treatments that supposedly contained ground horn from the mythical unicorn!

20

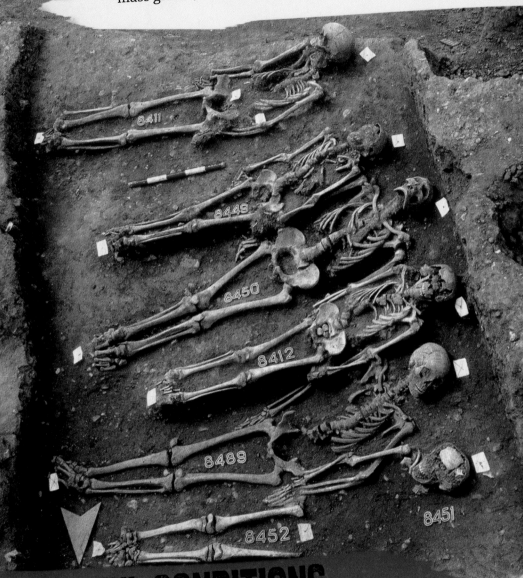

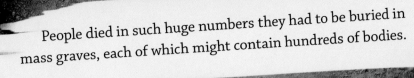

People died in such huge numbers they had to be buried in mass graves, each of which might contain hundreds of bodies.

8411

8449

8450

8412

8489

8452

8451

PITIFUL CONDITIONS

Boccaccio recorded conditions in cities: "The plight of the lower and most of the middle classes was even more pitiful to behold. Most of them remained in their houses, either through poverty or in hopes of safety, and fell sick by thousands. Since they received no care and attention, almost all of them died. Many . . . who died in their houses were only known to be dead because the neighbors smelled their decaying bodies."

Some people believed the Black Death was punishment from God and decided to perform **penance** in hopes God would take away the punishment. They marched barefoot throughout Europe whipping themselves with scourges, or sticks with spiked whips at one end. They were known as flagellants, and crowds gathered to watch them as they beat themselves and prayed for God's forgiveness.

The flagellants and many other Christians in Europe were **prejudiced** against Jews and believed Jews were causing the Black Death. They burned Jews at the stake or set fire to buildings filled with entire communities. Jews sometimes escaped the Black Death because they were forced to live isolated from the rest of society, but huge numbers were killed in these horrible ways by the time the plague ended.

The Deadly Details

The flagellants not only killed Jews, they also killed priests who spoke against their penance and other actions.

The pope tolerated the flagellants at first, but in October 1349, he ordered authorities to put a stop to them.

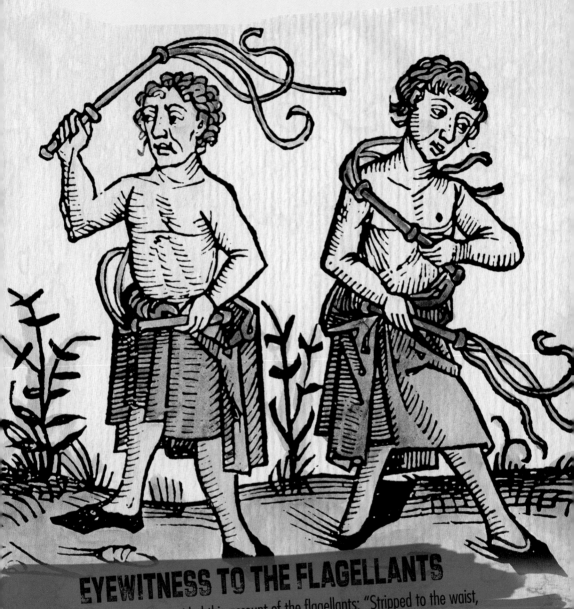

EYEWITNESS TO THE FLAGELLANTS

A French writer provided this account of the flagellants: "Stripped to the waist, they gathered in large groups and bands and marched in procession through the crossroads and squares of cities and good towns. They formed circles and beat upon their backs with weighted scourges, rejoicing as they did so in loud voices and singing hymns. ... They flogged their shoulders and arms, scourged with iron points so **zealously** as to draw blood."

EUROPE AFTER THE BLACK DEATH

By the time the Black Death ended, the staggering population loss led to economic problems. In cities, financial business was interrupted. People who owed money died, along with their family. People who had loaned money to others also died. Construction projects stopped for a while or were abandoned altogether. Craftsmen of all sorts had died, and there was no one to replace them. In the countryside, farms and entire villages died out or were abandoned. There was a shortage of labor to raise and harvest crops.

People also began to lose faith. They felt God had turned his back on them, so they turned away from religion. Wildly excited to be alive, they indulged in excessive eating and drinking, wore luxuriant clothing, and gambled.

The Deadly Details

An Italian historian writing about the plague included this sentence: "And the plague lasted until _____." He planned to fill in the blank after the plague ended, but he never got the chance—he died from plague in 1348.

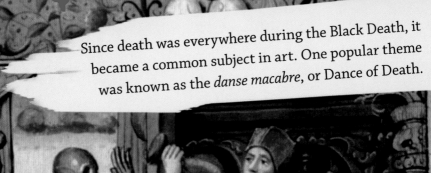

Since death was everywhere during the Black Death, it became a common subject in art. One popular theme was known as the *danse macabre*, or Dance of Death.

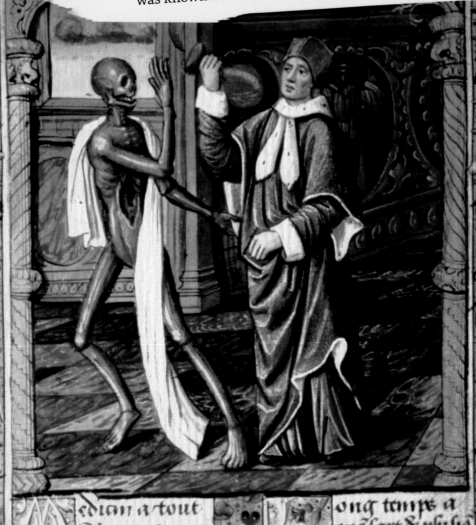

THE DANCE OF DEATH

The Black Death led to a theme called the Dance of Death in art. In paintings and printed images, the figure of Death appeared as a skeleton. Sometimes one or more skeletons were shown with living people going about their daily lives. Some pictures actually showed groups of skeletons dancing! All these images were reminders that death is always close at hand and a person might die at any time.

25

In spite of all this, a recent study found life improved after the Black Death. Survivors lived longer than people had lived before the disease appeared. Based on a study of bones, scientists found that after the Black Death, more than twice as many people lived past the age of 70. Why would that be?

It may be that the disease killed people who were weak and thus unlikely to live beyond age 70, so the survivors were stronger. Or it could have been survivors had a better diet. Historical records show people, especially the poor, were eating better after the Black Death. Available food had a smaller population to feed. Or perhaps it was a combination of the two. Strange that such a terrible event could yield something positive.

ThE DEadLy DEtaiLS

After the Black Death, survivors were eating more meat and fish and better-quality bread.

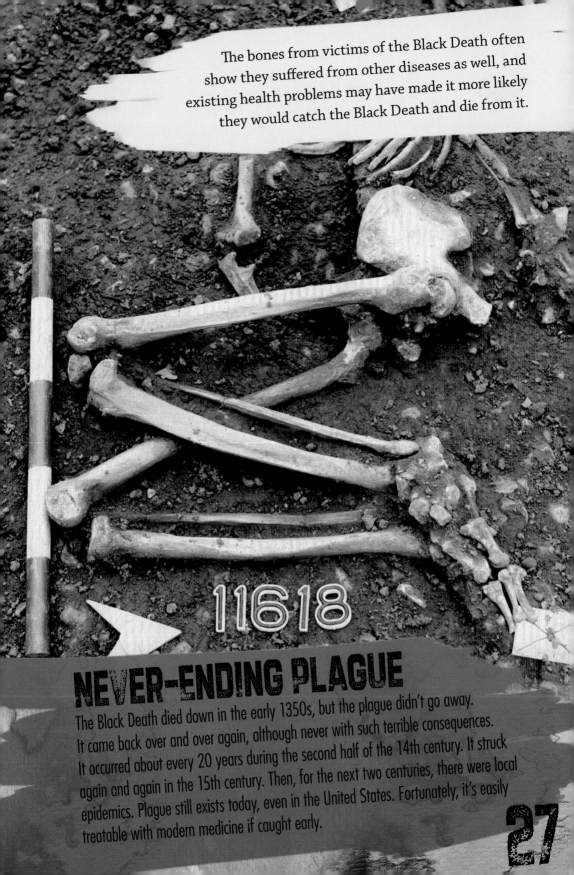

The bones from victims of the Black Death often show they suffered from other diseases as well, and existing health problems may have made it more likely they would catch the Black Death and die from it.

11618

NEVER-ENDING PLAGUE

The Black Death died down in the early 1350s, but the plague didn't go away. It came back over and over again, although never with such terrible consequences. It occurred about every 20 years during the second half of the 14th century. It struck again and again in the 15th century. Then, for the next two centuries, there were local epidemics. Plague still exists today, even in the United States. Fortunately, it's easily treatable with modern medicine if caught early.

MODERN RESEARCH ON THE BLACK DEATH

Because the Black Death was so terrible and the plague bacterium is alive and well, scientists continue to research it. Based on knowledge of the modern *Y. pestis* bacterium, some scientists doubt it could have caused the Black Death. But in 2000, a group of scientists found *Y. pestis* DNA in the teeth of Black Death victims.

Doubts continued. Then, recently, another group of scientists not only found *Y. pestis* DNA in the bones of Black Death victims, they also decoded its full genome.

Still, some scientists remain unconvinced *Y. pestis* was responsible for the Black Death. They believe a virus better explains the symptoms and the rate with which the disease spread. The arguments are likely to continue for some time.

The Deadly Details

One source of arguments over the cause of the Black Death is that some researchers in 2004 were unable to find any trace of *Y. pestis* DNA in teeth of the disease's victims.

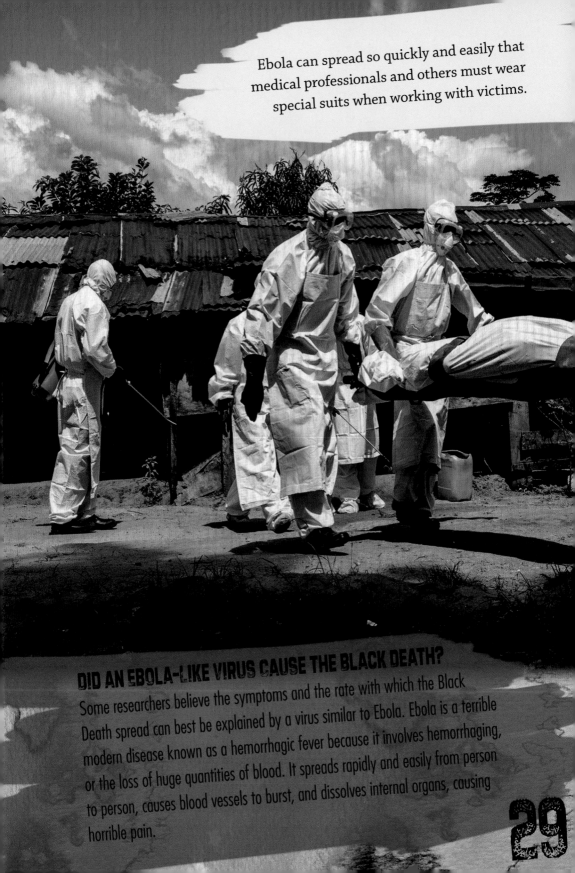

Ebola can spread so quickly and easily that medical professionals and others must wear special suits when working with victims.

DID AN EBOLA-LIKE VIRUS CAUSE THE BLACK DEATH?

Some researchers believe the symptoms and the rate with which the Black Death spread can best be explained by a virus similar to Ebola. Ebola is a terrible modern disease known as a hemorrhagic fever because it involves hemorrhaging, or the loss of huge quantities of blood. It spreads rapidly and easily from person to person, causes blood vessels to burst, and dissolves internal organs, causing horrible pain.

29

GLOSSARY

expire: to die

groin: the area between the lower part of the belly and the thigh

infection: the spread of germs, causing illness

isolate: to keep apart from others

lymph: pale liquid in the body that is part of the body's system for fighting infection

Mongol: one of the peoples of Mongolia who conquered much of Asia and eastern Europe in the 12th and 13th centuries

mucus: a thick slime produced by the body

penance: an act performed to show sorrow or to make amends for sins

prejudiced: having an unreasonable opinion of something or someone

pus: a thick, yellowish-white liquid formed in the body in response to infection

rodent: a small, furry animal with large front teeth, such as a mouse or rat

vomit: to throw up

zealously: feeling or showing strong and energetic support for something

FOR MORE INFORMATION

BOOKS

Jeffrey, Gary. *The Black Death*. New York, NY: Crabtree Publishing, 2014.

Senker, Cath. *The Black Death 1347–1350: The Plague Spreads Across Europe*. Chicago, IL: Raintree, 2006.

Zahler, Diane. *The Black Death*. Minneapolis, MN: Twenty-First Century Books, 2009.

WEBSITES

The Black Death
www.sciencemuseum.org.uk/broughttolife/themes/diseases/black_death.aspx
Learn more about the Black Death and people's attempts to deal with it on this interactive website.

The Black Death
historymedren.about.com/od/theblackdeath/p/blackdeath.htm
Read more about the Black Death, and learn about its effects on society in the 1300s.

Plague: The Black Death
science.nationalgeographic.com/science/health-and-human-body/human-diseases/plague-article/
Read a brief history of plague, and learn about the types of plague and where plague exists today.

INDEX